Claudien Uwanyirigira

Determinants of pregnancy desire in HIV-positive women

Claudien Uwanyirigira

Determinants of pregnancy desire in HIV-positive women

ScienciaScripts

Imprint

Any brand names and product names mentioned in this book are subject to trademark, brand or patent protection and are trademarks or registered trademarks of their respective holders. The use of brand names, product names, common names, trade names, product descriptions etc. even without a particular marking in this work is in no way to be construed to mean that such names may be regarded as unrestricted in respect of trademark and brand protection legislation and could thus be used by anyone.

Cover image: www.ingimage.com

This book is a translation from the original published under ISBN 978-613-8-40975-5.

Publisher:
Sciencia Scripts
is a trademark of
Dodo Books Indian Ocean Ltd. and OmniScriptum S.R.L publishing group

120 High Road, East Finchley, London, N2 9ED, United Kingdom
Str. Armeneasca 28/1, office 1, Chisinau MD-2012, Republic of Moldova, Europe
Printed at: see last page
ISBN: 978-620-6-02820-8

TABLE OF CONTENTS

DEDICATION

To God Almighty

To my late parents, brothers and sisters

To our Dear Wife Laurence UWITONZE

To our children, Gaël.Gretta and Ghita

Dear Sisters,

My friends and acquaintances

This brief is dedicated to

FOREWORD

This work is the fruit of long and hard efforts.

However, these efforts would have been in vain, if we had not benefited from the assistance of several people to whom we owe a debt of gratitude forever.

Our thanks go to the Rwandan Government who, through the Ministry of Health, granted me a scholarship through the GF Project Management Unit.

Our thanks also go to the faculty of the UNR School of Public Health for the great effort they have put into our work throughout our supervision.

A particular homage is addressed to Professor Cyprien MUNYANSHONGORE, Director of the thesis, who despite his multiple preoccupations, accepted without difficulty to guide our research. He was always ready to devote himself to us. May his attitudes, his advice and his scientific rigor, so constructive, find their fruit here.

I would like to thank the health personnel of the Musha, Nyagasambu, Munyaga and Nzige health centers and those of the Rwamagana Hospital working in the VCT/PMTCT and ARVs departments.

We also feel indebted to our dear wife and children who have endured our absence, depriving themselves of our important affection

To you, dear colleagues, first cohort of the Master of Public Health, evening program, for your accompaniment, and your technical and moral support

Finally, I would like to express my deepest gratitude to all the other people who, from near or far, have contributed to the realization of this work

Claudien UWANYIRIGIRA

SUMMARY

The AIDS epidemic continues to worsen around the world and is a real public health problem.

In industrialized countries in the United States, Australia, and France, the prevalence of pregnancy among HIV-positive women who were informed of their HIV status and receiving ARVs ranged from 18% to 40%. 69% of these women wanted to have one or more children in the future.

In Cameroon, in Yaoundé, one-third of 40 HIV-positive men and women who responded to the questionnaire reported having unprotected sex, the main reasons given being the desire to have a child or the refusal of the partner to use a barrier method.

This problem is of concern in Rwanda and in particular in Rwamagana District where we conducted our study on the determinants of desire for pregnancy among HIV positive women under antiretroviral treatment.

The study hypothesis is: The proportion of repeat pregnancies as well as motherhood and desire for children among HIV-positive women on antiretroviral therapy is high in Rwamagana District.

In order to do this, the following objectives have been set:

- Determine the proportion of pregnancies among HIV-positive women

- Determine the proportion of HIV-infected women who want more children in the future

- Identify factors that determine the desire to have children after being subjected to antiretroviral drugs

- To determine the level of knowledge of HIV-positive women about the usefulness of contraceptive methods to reduce the risk of mother-to-child transmission

- To assess the attitude of health care personnel regarding messages to be given to HIV-positive women on ARVs regarding the desire for pregnancy.

To achieve these objectives, a descriptive cross-sectional study was conducted among 260 HIV-infected women on ARVs and followed up in health facilities with VCT/PMTCT services and ARVs.

The main findings of the study are:

26.9% of the women in our study became pregnant after being informed of their HIV positive status

38.5% of HIV positive women on ARVs want to have children in the future. Apart from other considerations on the desire for motherhood i.e. trust in ARVs, fear of in-laws, HIV-negative status of the previous child etc., there is no evidence that the desire to have a child is a major factor in the decision to have children.

This desire is also motivated by age, parity and regular use of contraceptives.

82.7% of the women in our study know the importance of using contraceptives while 76.9% know the importance of using ARVs during pregnancy and delivery to reduce the risk of mother-to-child transmission.

Thus, the results of our study show that HIV-positive women became pregnant after being informed of their serological status (26.9%) and a significant proportion of HIV-positive women undergoing antiretroviral treatment want to have children in the future for various reasons (38.5%).

Finally, involving men more in FP programs, VCT/PMTCT services, in order to help couples with their reproductive health, and strengthening the integration of reproductive health and FP activities into HIV/AIDS services (PMTCT, HIV counseling and testing, and management of HIV-positive patients) could partially solve these problems.

CHAPTER 1: INTRODUCTION

1.1. Presentation of the problem

1.1.1. Definitions of concepts

1.1.1.1 HIV

HIV, the human immunodeficiency virus, is the virus that causes AIDS in humans. At present, two types of virus are known: HIV-1 and HIV-2. Both types of virus are responsible for identical clinical manifestations and can infect a person concomitantly; however, HIV-1 is more virulent and more frequent in sub-Saharan Africa **(1)**

1.1.1.2 AIDS

The acronym AIDS stands for Acquired Immunodeficiency Syndrome. It is the advanced stage of HIV infection during which the infected person presents opportunistic infections and a disturbed biological balance **(2)**

1.1.1.3 HIV and pregnancy

There is no faster progression of the disease, but it should be noted that the CD4 rate decreases, but this is explained by the increase in the volume of distribution related to the pregnancy of the placenta and the amniotic fluid, which causes the CD4 rate to be lowered; on the other hand, the risk of opportunistic infection exists if there is an immune deficiency **(3)**.

Today, pregnancy has a real place in the life of an HIV-positive woman without jeopardizing her health. Since AIDS has become a chronic disease, women with the disease want to live their femininity and have a normal sexuality. The desire to have children when she is of childbearing age is a natural consequence **(4)**.

1.1.1.4 HIV and anti-retroviral treatment in pregnant women Pregnancies in women under anti-retroviral treatment are increasingly frequent and two situations can be envisaged, when :

- the treatment received prior to pregnancy is effective and well tolerated if the immunovirological results are satisfactory (CD4 > 350/mm3 and the viral load is < 5000 copies/ml) and stable.

Whatever treatment is continued during pregnancy, AZT should be administered at the time of delivery by intravenous infusion and then to the newborn during the first weeks of life **(5)**.

- the treatment received prior to pregnancy is ineffective if the immunoviral results are not satisfactory (CD4<350/mm3 and viral load >5000 copies/ml) despite good compliance, a change in antiretroviral treatment is desirable**(5-6)**.

1.1.2 Formulation of the problem

The number of people living with HIV worldwide is estimated at 33,245,000.HIV infection has caused the death of more than 20 million people since the first case of acquired immunodeficiency syndrome(AIDS) was identified in 1981.In 2007 alone, UNAIDS estimates 2,500,000 new HIV-related infections and 2,100,000 AIDS-related deaths. The proportion of women among infected adults has gradually increased to stabilize around 50% ά from the 1990s**(7)**

In 2003, an estimated 40 million people worldwide had the human immunodeficiency virus (HIV) or acquired immunodeficiency syndrome (AIDS), including approximately 37 million adults and 2.5 million children**(7)**.

Women account for about half of these cases **(7-8)**.

This proportion is worrisome since the majority of HIV infections in children are acquired perinatally.

In Canada, an estimated 7,700 women were living with HIV at the end of 2002**(8)**. According to 2005 surveillance data, women account for approximately one-quarter of reported positive HIV tests**(8-9)**.

Mother-to-child transmission of HIV is estimated to account for more than 95% of pediatric HIV infections in sub-Saharan Africa.

Almost 90% of HIV-infected children live in sub-Saharan Africa **(8)**, because since the beginning of the HIV/AIDS epidemic, sub-Saharan Africa has always been one of the regions most severely affected by HIV infection **(9-10)**

In Rwanda in 2005, the number of PLWHA was 147,234 of which 62,147 (42.8%) were men and 85,102 (57.8) were women. Of these women 13,872 (16.3%) were pregnant.

Thus, a study by Birungi on the determinants of HIV-positive women's desire to become pregnant in Gicumbi District showed that 21.6% of the women surveyed became pregnant after being informed of their HIV-positive status **(2)**.

In light of the above, we wondered why HIV-positive women who receive sufficient counseling information while attending VCT/PMTCT and ARV'S services continue to desire new pregnancies.

For this reason, we focused our study in Rwamagana District to determine the reasons why HIV-positive women who have been on antiretroviral treatment become pregnant.

1.1.3 Interest of the subject

1.1.3.1 Personal interest

Realizing that the reports that come from our health facilities, where comprehensive care for people living with HIV is operational, we have observed that in some health centers in Rwamagana District, during our supervisions, a large number of HIV-positive women who attend VCT/PMTCT and ARV services become pregnant again, even though they have been informed of their seroprevalence and in spite of the advice they receive during counseling not to conceive.

As a result, the prevalence of mother-to-child transmission is becoming increasingly high. No intermediate option is given to them in the sense that they want to have children or when they are prevented from having them.

This situation has awakened us to be able to identify the proportion of women who wish to have children, being HIV positive and on ARV's and the factors that motivate these repeated pregnancies, in all the Health Centers with VCT/PMTCT and ARV's services in Rwamagana District

1.1.3.2 Scientific interest

Studies show that many HIV-positive women want to have children and do have children even after knowing their HIV-positive status.

The present study will allow us to determine the proportion of HIV-positive women who wish to have children, the confidence attributed to ARVs that can reduce the risk of mother-to-child transmission, and the different factors that encourage these women to undergo so-called repeat pregnancies while on ARV treatment.

This work could also serve as a reference for other researchers to guide their work in this area.

1.1.4. Description of the study environment

The District of Rwamagana, created in January 2006, is one of the seven Districts that make up the Eastern Province, of which it is the capital. It was created by merging the former Districts of Muhazi, Bicumbi, two sectors of Gasabo (Fumbwe and Mununu), three sectors of Kabarondo (Kaduha, Rweru and Nkungu) and the municipality of Rwamagana. It is composed of 14 sectors, 82 cells and 474 villages and covers an area of 691.6 km^2 .

It is bordered to the south by the District of Ngoma, to the north by the Districts of Gatsibo and Gicumbi, to the east by the District of Kayonza, and to the west by the Districts of Gasabo, Kicukiro and Bugesera.

Rwamagana District has a total population of 2,223,653 distributed among 4,8754 households with an average density of 323 inhabitants with 78% of households living in villages/umudugudu.

Relief:

Its relief is characterized by plateaus whose altitude varies between 1400 and 1700m. The general configuration of the relief is constituted by an uplift in altitude from the East and a notable lowering of the mini plateaus in ridges oriented towards Lake Muhazi in the North and Lake Mugesera in the South.

Climate:

Rwamagana District has a moderate tropical climate that is often humid with a tendency á aridity. It has four seasons:two rainy seasons and two dry seasons. The average temperature between 19 and 30° C is constant throughout the year. The average rainfall is around 1000mm.

Socio-economic situation:

With agri-livestock farming as the main economic activity, where more than 80% of the population lives from traditional farming, demographic pressure and scattered settlements significantly reduce the amount of land available for farming. More than 95% of the population uses traditional farming tools (hoes, machetes, etc.). Most of them use organic fertilizer because chemical fertilizer is only timidly introduced.

Beans are the most produced and serve as a staple food, with the annual harvest in 2006 estimated at 4,644,531 kg. Other important crops are sorghum, corn, sweet potatoes, potatoes and cassava, and bananas. Rice is grown in the swamps.

Given its proximity to the city of Kigali, agricultural production is sold in markets located in almost all sectors and benefits from buyers coming from Kigali. In order to curb the problems of stock shortages and ensure food security, systematic and compulsory storage strategies have been put in place and storage silos are operational throughout the district.

In addition to coffee and tomato, other industrial crops are being introduced such as chili, Moringa, vanilla and Macadamia. Efforts are being made to popularize these crops which can generate much more income and thus accelerate the economic development of the population of the district.

Large and small livestock are also raised, but this is not well developed, with daily milk production in 2006 estimated at an average of 11,702 liters, of which only 4,466 liters (38%) were sold.

Currently, extensive livestock farming is tending to disappear in favor of permanent stall farming. In 2006, the district's cattle population consisted of 21,958 cows, of which 16,542 were of the "ankole" breed (73.3%), 3,460 were of the hybrid breed, and 1,956 were modern cows. In addition to cows, there are goats, sheep, pigs, chickens, rabbits, etc. A few farms can be found in certain areas.

The presence of lakes Muhazi and Mugesera favors fishing and constitutes an important economic potential.

Rwamagana District (in the former Muhazi) is rich in precious stones: Cassiterite, Colombo tantalum and Wolfram which are exploited by the Régie des Mines du Rwanda (REDEMI) and exported to Europe. Besides these precious stones, it also has quarries for building stones, sand, clay, and laterite for the construction and maintenance of houses and roads.

In Rwamagana District, there is a small processing unit (IHUMURE) for the production of wine and fruit juices and the construction of a unit for the treatment of Kaolin for the production of paints has been completed.

There are a few artisans practicing different trades in the center of Rwamagana.

With regard to the standard of living of the various segments of the population, it should be noted that the majority of the population derives its income mainly from the sale of agricultural products. According to Ubudehe's data, the Rwamagana district has social categories ranging from the poorest (abatindi nyakujya) to the richest (abakire).

The Rwamagana District has not been sheltered from the effects of the genocide and has many children orphaned by the genocide, widows and widowers who need assistance. In total, there are nearly 12,673 genocide survivors, of whom 5,576 are vulnerable, or 44%.

Health status:

From a health point of view, the following diseases are the main causes of morbidity:

> Malaria is the leading cause of morbidity and mortality (39% of proportional morbidity)

> Acute Respiratory Infections

> Skin conditions

> HIV/AIDS

> Intestinal parasitosis

The main health indicators showing the current situation in Rwamagana District are as follows

> Vaccination coverage: 97.6%.

> Assisted delivery at the CS/Hospital: 60%.

> Family planning: 10%.

> Utilization rate of curative services: 63.6

Within the framework of the fight against HIV/AIDS, the situation at the district level is as follows

> 8/11 health centers have VCT/PMTCT services

> 6 health centers (Munyaga, Nyagasambu, Karenge Nzige, Rubona and Musha), and the hospital have ARV services

> 1Private clinic (AVEGA) has a VCT/ARVs service

> The HIV/AIDS prevalence rate in 2007 was 5.8% (people tested in health facilities)

The 3 health facilities have only VCT/PMTCT services and only one does not have these three services at all (this is the Nyakariro Health Center).

1.1.5 Review of the literature

According to UNAIDS (Joint United Nations Programme on HIV/AIDS) and WHO (World Health Organization), an estimated 2.5 (2.2-2.6) million children under the age of 15 were living with HIV in 2007(**19**). 420,000 (350,000-540,000) children are thought to have been infected with HIV during 2007, accounting for about 17% of the 2.5 (1.8-4.1) million new infections that occurred during the year(**19**).

In industrialized countries, in the United States, Australia and France, the prevalence of pregnancy among HIV-positive women informed of their serostatus and receiving ARVs varies between 18%-40%. 69% of these women wanted to have one or more children in the future.

Almost 90% of HIV-infected children live in sub-Saharan Africa (**16**).

Mother-to-child transmission of HIV is estimated to account for more than 95% of pediatric HIV infections in sub-Saharan Africa.

In Cameroon, in Yaoundé, one-third of 40 HIV-positive men and women responding to a questionnaire reported having unprotected sex. The main reasons given were the desire to have a child or the refusal of the partner to use a barrier method (8).

Studies in Uganda (12), Zambia (11), and the United States of America (10) reported that 7%, 22%, and 29% of HIV-positive women respectively wanted new births.

Two earlier studies in Rwanda reported the percentage of HIV+ women who wanted new pregnancies as ranging from 8% to 40% (23).

In addition, a study by Birungi found that 21.6% of subjects in his study became pregnant after being informed of their HIV+ status (2).

The question remains as to why these women are pregnant when they have been informed of the possibility of transmission of the virus (HIV) from mother to child and have been advised not to become pregnant again.

1.1.6. Hypothesis and objectives of the study

1.1.6.1 Hypothesis

The proportion of repeat pregnancies as well as childbearing and desire for children among HIV-positive women on antiretroviral treatment is high in Rwamagana District. This situation is explained by:

1. Confidence in antiretrovirals, having HIV-negative children despite their HIV status

2. HIV-positive women's lack of knowledge about the usefulness of contraceptive methods to reduce the risk of mother-to-child transmission

3. Influence of socio-cultural factors

4. Indifference of health personnel to the key messages to be given to HIV-positive women on ARVs

1.1.6.2 Objectives

1.1.6.2.1 General objective

Our study aims to analyze the determinants of pregnancy desire in HIV-positive women undergoing antiretroviral treatment, in order to contribute to the reduction of mother-to-child transmission of the virus.

1.1.6.2.2 Specific objectives

The specific objectives of this study are to:

1.	Determine the proportion of pregnancies among HIV-positive women

2.	Determine the proportion of HIV-infected women who want more children in the future

3.	Identify factors determining the desire to have children after being subjected to Antiretrovirals

4.	To determine the level of knowledge of HIV-positive women about the usefulness of contraceptive methods to reduce the risk of transmission from mother á child

5.	To assess the attitude of health care staff regarding messages to be given to HIV-positive women on ARVs regarding the desire for pregnancy.

CHAPTER 2: MATERIALS AND METHODS

11.1. TYPE OF STUDY :

Our study is of the cross-sectional type with a descriptive aim. It was carried out among HIV-infected women on ARVs and followed up in health facilities within the framework of PMTCT, in Fosa with VCT/PMTCT services and ARVs in Rwamagana District

11.2 VARIABLES

11.2.1 Dependent variables

Desire for motherhood after being on antiretroviral treatment

11.2.2 Independent variables:

Age, parity, education level of the wife, education level of the husband, marital status, knowledge of the husband's HIV status, number of children or pregnancies among HIV-positive women, number of HIV-infected women wanting more children in the future, reasons for wanting to have children after being on antiretroviral drugs. Use of contraceptive methods, intention to use contraceptive methods in the future; reasons for not using contraception in an HIV-positive woman, knowledge of VCT/PMTCT& ARV service approaches, knowledge of the benefits of using ARVs during pregnancy or childbirth, and the place or services that inform them about the benefits of using ARVs.

11.3 . Analysis Plan :

To test our hypothesis and achieve our specific objectives, we proceeded as follows:

1. To determine the proportion of pregnancies among HIV-positive women, we asked which women had children or became pregnant after knowing their HIV-positive status and determined their proportion.

2. To determine the proportion of HIV-infected women who want more children in the future, we asked which HIV-positive women on ARVs wanted to have one or more children.

3. To identify the factors that determine the desire to have children after being on antiretroviral therapy, we asked about the reasons that led or are leading them to want children.

4. To determine the level of knowledge of HIV-positive women on the usefulness of contraceptive methods to reduce the risk of mother-to-child transmission, we asked women who use contraceptive methods if they know the benefits of using contraceptive methods and taking ARVs during pregnancy and delivery in reducing mother-to-child

14

transmission of the virus

5. To assess the attitude of health care staff toward giving key messages to HIV-infected women on antiretroviral therapy to avoid new pregnancies, we asked health care staff what type of message they give during counseling and what barriers they face if the attitude was deemed negative.

For all these variables, the search for association was done using the Chi-square test. To investigate the significance of the independent variables associated with the dependent variable, we used logistic regression. Significant association was assessed by Wald chi-square.

11.4 Sampling

II 4.1. Sample size and sample selection

■ **Sample size calculation**

To calculate our sample size, we used the following formula: **n=** $\dfrac{E^2 \times p(1-p)}{i^2}$

With n=Sample **size**

E2= is the value of the normal variable centered reduced which corresponds to the value of the probability for a confidence interval fixed at 95%= 1.96

p is the prevalence of desire for motherhood in our study population, as Gicumbi District has almost the same epidemiological characteristic as Rwamagana District, we will use the data found in Gicumbi by Birungi , i.e., 21.6% of women became pregnant after being informed of their á HIV status.

i is a precision with a tolerable error margin of 5%.

1-p is the absence of desire for motherhood in the study population

Thus, **n** was equal to $\dfrac{(1.96)^2 \times 0{,}216 \times 0{,}784}{(0.05)^2} = 260$ Women

260 people were surveyed. For each selected health facility, at least 52 people were fully interviewed, but not more than 55 subjects. The interviews will be administered progressively until the number of subjects to be interviewed per facility is reached.

■ **Sample selection**

The persons included in this study were HIV-infected women, on ARV, attending PMTCT, VCT and ARV services at Rwamagana Hospital and in Musha, Nyagasambu, Nzige and

Munyaga Health Centers offering the above services (i.e., 2 Public Health Centers, 2 Agreed Health Centers and one Hospital).

The women to be interviewed met the following criteria:

Be at least 18 years old; voluntarily agree to participate á the survey, have become pregnant and or have at least one child after being followed by the health facility in the context of PMTCT, have started ARVs at the time of data collection.

The respondents were recruited during ANC or postnatal visits to the health facilities for their medical follow-up and/or for the follow-up of their children, or after the counseling services offered to these women. Each participant was interviewed once.

11.5. Material:

The data collection took place in June 2009 and the information was collected through a questionnaire that we developed. The data entry and analysis will be done using SPSS 12.0.1 and the text was written using Word. The results were present after a univariate analysis and to determine the associations between the variables, a bivariate analysis was done. The chi-square test was used to determine if there was an association between the variables in the study in order to compare the proportions. Multivariate analysis was used to determine the strength of association of the independent variables and desire for pregnancy. The significance level considered was 5%.

11.6. Use of the results obtained

The results of our study will be used by decision makers in Rwamagana District and the Ministry of Health in particular to :

Strengthen the integration of reproductive health and FP activities into HIV/AIDS services (PMTCT, HIV counseling and testing, and care of HIV-positive patients).

J Set up a follow-up program for HIV-positive couples who wish to have children to enable them to have pregnancies in the best conditions in order to reduce vertical transmission

To awaken health personnel to be able to provide quality services to women and men who attend VCT, PMTCT&ARV services in order to enable them to have all the necessary information on reducing vertical transmission and preventing unwanted pregnancies.

J To explore the influence of ARV treatment on the contraceptive practice and reproductive life of PLHIV.

CHAPTER 3: RESULTS

III.1.SOCIO-DEMOGRAPHIC CHARACTERISTICS OF THE STUDY SUBJECTS

Age:

The age of the women enrolled in our study ranged from 19 to 48 years. 46.2% were under 35 years of age, and 53.8% were over 35 years of age. The average age is 33.6 years. **Educational level of the women:**

36.5% of the women in our study have completed elementary school, while those who have never attended school represent 26.9%.

17.3% attended but did not complete primary school, 15.3% attended or completed secondary school, and very few women in our sample, 3.8%, attended university.

Husband's education level:

The majority of the partners of the women in our sample, 61.5%, had completed elementary school, 15.3% had attended but not completed elementary school, and 11.5% had attended or completed secondary school.

9.6% have never been to school and 1.9% have attended university.

Woman's occupation:

About 67.3% of the women in our sample do housework and agricultural work, 25% have paid work and 7.6% do housework only.

Husband's occupation:

78.8% of the women partners in our study are farmers, 13.4% have a paid job and 7.6% have no known profession.

Marital status of the woman:

The women in our study who are legally married represent 44.2% and 23% are widows and 19.2% are single mothers.

7.6% are divorced while 5.7% are separated.

Parity:

80.8% of our study have at least one child and 19.2% have no children.

The elements described above are represented in Table 1.

Table 1: Sociodemographic characteristics of the study population

Features	Frequency	Percentage
Age (in years)		
<35	120	46,2
> 35	140	53,8
Total	**260**	
Woman's level of education		
No studies done	70	26,9
Primary education attended and not completed	45	17,3
Primary education completed	95	36,5
Secondary education attended/completed	40	15,3
Higher education attended/completed	10	3,8
Total	**260**	
Husband's level of education		
No studies done	25	9,6
Primary education attended and not completed	40	15,3
Primary education completed	160	61,5
Secondary education attended/completed	30	11,5
Higher education attended/completed	5	1,9
Total	**260**	
Woman's occupation		
Household and agricultural work Household work only	175	67,3
Paid work	20	7,6
	65	25
Total	**260**	
Profession of the husband		
Agri-breeder	205	78,8
Paid work	35	13,4
No known occupation	20	7,6
Total	**260**	

Marital status of the woman		
	50	
	115	
	60	19,2 44,2 23
Single mother Married	20	7,6
Widow Divorced Separated	15	5,7
Total	**260**	
Parity		
No children	50	19.2
At least one child	210	80.8
Total	**260**	

111.2. Actual results

111.2.1 Frequency of pregnancy after knowledge of HIV status

111.2.1.1 Proportion of women who became pregnant after being informed of their HIV-positive status

26.9% of women had at least one child after being informed of their status

HIV positive and 73.1% did not have children.

Table 2 shows this.

Table 2: Distribution of women by whether they became pregnant or

not after being informed of their HIV-positive status.

Variable	Workforce	Percentage
No children	190	73,1
At least one child	70	26,9
Total	260	100

III.2.1.2 Influential relationship between selected study variables and becoming pregnant after being informed of one's HIV-positive status.

Age:

Among women under 35 years of age, 29.1% became pregnant after being informed of their HIV-positive status, and among women 35 years of age and older, 25% became pregnant after being informed of their HIV-positive status.

There was no statistical association between being pregnant and the woman's age (p=0.435).

Woman's education level:

For women with primary education and no schooling, 31.8% became pregnant after being informed of their HIV-positive status and 23.3% of women who became pregnant after being informed of their HIV-positive status had completed elementary school and above.

There was no statistical association between being pregnant after being informed of HIV-positive status and the woman's education level (p=0.691).

Husband's education level:

For women whose husbands attended primary school and below, 26.6% became pregnant after being informed of their HIV-positive status, and for women whose husbands attended secondary school and above, 28.5% became pregnant after being informed of their HIV-positive status.

There was no statistical association between becoming pregnant after being informed of HIV status and the husband's education level (P=0.403).

Woman's occupation:

For women engaged in household and agricultural work, 27.1% became pregnant after being informed of their HIV+ status; and for women in other occupations, 20% became pregnant after being informed of their HIV positive status.

There was no statistical association between becoming pregnant after being informed of HIV status and the woman's occupation (p=0.777).

Marital status of the woman:

Among women who are married, 26% became pregnant after being informed of their HIV-positive status and 27.5% of women with other marital status became pregnant after being informed of their HIV-positive status.

There was no statistical association between becoming pregnant after being informed of HIV-positive status and the woman's marital status(p=0.308). **Parity:**

For women without children, 40% became pregnant after being informed of their HIV-positive status, and for those with at least one child, 23.8% became pregnant after being informed of their HIV-positive status.

There was no statistical association between becoming pregnant after being informed of

HIV-positive status and parity (p=0.460).

The elements described above are represented in Table 3.

Table 3: Influential relationship between selected study variables and becoming pregnant after being informed of one's HIV-positive status.

Variable	Workforce	Percentage of women who had at least one child after knowing their HIV+ status	Those who have not been pregnant	X^2	p	Decision
Age of the woman (in years)						
< 35	120			48.956	0.435	NS
> 35	140	29,1(35) 25(35)	70,8(85) 75(105)			
Total	260	26,9(70)	73(190)			
Woman's level of education						
Primary attended but not completed + no school	110	31,8(35)	68,2(75)	3.896	0.691	NS
Primary completed and up	150	23,3(35)	76,6(115)			
Total	260	26,9 (70)	73(190)			
Husband's level of education	225	26,6(60)	73,3(165)			
Primary education and less Secondary education and more	35	28,5(10)	71,4 (25)	8,32	0,403	NS
Total	260	26,9 (70)	73(190)			
Woman's occupation						
Household and agricultural work	240			6,441	0,777	NS
Other	20	27,1(65) 20(5)	72,9(175) 75(15)			
Total	260	26,9(70)	73(190)			
Marital status						
Brides	115	26(30)	73,9(85)	9,420	0,308	NS
Other	145	27,5(40)	72,9 (105)			
Total	260	26,9(70)	73(190)			
Parity						
No children	50	40(20)		5,68	0,460	NS
At least one child	210	23,8(50)				
Total	260	26,9(70)				

III.2.2 Proportion of HIV-positive women on antiretroviral treatment who wish to have children in the future

III.2.2.1 Proportion of HIV-positive women on antiretroviral treatment who wish to have children in the future

Overall, 38.5% of HIV-positive women on antiretroviral therapy said they wanted more children, while 61.5% did not.

Table 4 shows this.

Table 4: Proportion of women on antiretroviral treatment who want to have children in the future

Variable	Workforce	Percentage
Desire to have children		
Yes	100	38,5
No	160	61.5
TOTAL	**260**	**100**

111.2.2.2 . Factors determining the desire for motherhood among HIV-positive women on ARVs according to reasons.

170 women, or 65.3% of the subjects in our study, gave their reasons for becoming pregnant despite their HIV+ status.

The first reason is the confidence attributed to ARVs which was raised by 38% of the women, followed by the HIV-negative status of the previous child at 17.6%, the refusal of the husband to use condoms and the husband's desire to have a child at 14.7%, 8% reported that they need a replacement, and the simple pleasure of having a child and the fear of the in-laws were cited at 2.9% each.

Table 5 shows this.

Variables	Workforce	percentage
Factors determining the desire for motherhood among HIV-positive women on antiretroviral therapy		
1. I trust ARVs	65	38
2. I am afraid of the in-laws	5	2,9
3. The previous child is negative	30	17,6
4. For the simple pleasure of having a child	5	2,9

5. If I don't give birth, others will laugh at me	0	0
6. My husband wants it	25	14,7
7. I need a replacement	15	8,8
8. My husband refuses to use a condom	25	14,7
9. We are a discordant couple	O	0
TOTAL	**170**	**100**

111.2.2.3   Other factors that influence the desire for motherhood in HIV-positive women after they have been on antiretroviral therapy

Age:

Among women aged 35 and over, 39% want to have children in the future and among women under 35, 37.5% want to have children in the future.

There is a statistical relationship between the desire to have children in HIV-positive women on antiretroviral treatment and the age of the woman (p=0.000)

Woman's education level:

For women who have attended primary school but did not finish it+no school, 42.7% want to have children in the future and for women who have finished elementary school and >, 35.3% want to have children.

There was no statistical association between the desire for motherhood in HIV-positive women on antiretroviral treatment and the woman's level of education (p=0.172).

Husband's education level:

For women whose husbands have attended secondary school and above, 50% of women want to have children in the future and for women whose husbands have attended primary school and below, 36.3% want to have children.

There was no statistical relationship between the desire for motherhood in HIV-positive women on antiretroviral treatment and the husband's level of education (p=0.325).

Profession:

For women who are involved in other activities, 50% want to have children in the future, while 37.5% of women who do housework and agricultural work express a desire to have children in the future.

There was no statistical relationship between the desire for motherhood in HIV-positive women on antiretroviral treatment and their occupation (p=0.518).

Marital status:

For women who are married, 39.1% want to have children in the future and for women with another marital status, 37.9% express a desire to have children in the future.

There was no statistical relationship between the desire for motherhood in HIV-positive women on antiretroviral therapy and their marital status (p=0.302).

Parity:

For women who have no children, 60% want to have children in the future and for those who have at least one child, 34% want to have children in the future.

There is a statistical relationship between the desire for motherhood in HIV-positive women undergoing antiretroviral treatment and parity (p=0.04).

Knowledge of husband's HIV status by the wife: For women who do not know the HIV status of their husbands/partners, 53% want to have children and 32% of women who know the HIV status of their husbands/partners want to have children in the future.

There was no statistical association between the desire for motherhood in HIV-positive women undergoing antiretroviral treatment and the wife's knowledge of the husband's HIV status (p=0.125).

Regular or no use of contraceptive methods:

For women who regularly use contraceptives, 39% want to have children in the future and for those who do not regularly use these methods, 37.9% want to have children in the future.

There is a statistical relationship between the desire for childbearing in HIV-positive women on antiretroviral therapy and regular contraceptive use (p=0.000). The elements described above are presented in Table 6.

Table 6: Influence of selected variables in our study on desire for childbearing among HIV-positive women after receiving antiretroviral therapy.

Variable	Workforce	Percentage of women on ARVs who want to have children	Those who do not wish to have children	X^2	P	Decision
Age of the woman (in years)	120	37,5(45)	62,5(75)			
< 35	140	39,2(55)	60,7(85)	18,904	0,000	***

> 35	260	38,5(100)	61,5(160)			
Total						
Woman's level of education Primary attended but not completed + no school Primary completed and above **Total**	110 150 **260**	42,7(47) 35,3 (53) **38,5 (100)**	57,3(63) 64,6(97) **61,5(160)**	4,997	0,072	NS
Husband's level of education Primary education and less Secondary education and more **Total**	220 40 **260**	36,3(80) 50(20) **38,5 (100)**	63,6(140) 50(20) **61,5(160)**	4,653	0,325	NS
Woman's occupation Household and agricultural work Other **Total**	240 20 **260**	37,5(90) 50(10) **38,5(100)**	62,5(150) 50(10) **61,5(160)**	4,221	0,518	NS
Marital status Brides Other Total	115 145 260	39,1(45) 37,9(55) **38,5(100)**	60,8(70) 62,1(90) **61,5(160)**	4,862	0,302	NS
Parity No children At least one child Total	50 210 **260**	60 (30) 33 (70) **38,5(100)**	(20) (140) **61,5(160)**	8,802	0,04	*
Wife's knowledge of husband's HIV status Know Do not know Total	185 75 260	32(60) 53(40) **38,5(100)**	67,5(70) 46,6,1(90) **61,5(160)**	5,70	0,125	NS
Regular or no contraceptive use Use Do not use Total	115 145 260	39(45) 37,9(55) **38,5(100)**	60,8(70) 62,1(90) **61,5(160)**	0,51	0,000	***

III.2.4 Knowledge of HIV-positive women about the importance of using contraceptive methods and ARVs during pregnancy and delivery to reduce the risk of mother-to-child transmission

III.2.4.1 HIV-positive women's knowledge of the usefulness of contraceptive methods to reduce the risk of transmission from mother to child

82.7% of women know the importance of using contraceptives in reducing transmission and 17.3% do not know this usefulness

III.2.4.2 Knowledge of HIV-positive women on the importance of using ARVs during pregnancy and delivery to reduce the risk of transmission from mother to child

76.9% of women know the importance of using ARVs during pregnancy and delivery to reduce the risk of mother-to-child transmission and 23.1% do not.

Table 7 shows this.

<u>Table 7</u>: Knowledge of HIV-positive women on ARVs about the importance of using contraceptive methods and taking ARVs during pregnancy and childbirth to reduce the risk of mother-to-child transmission

Variables	Workforce	Percentage
Knowledge of the usefulness of using contraceptive methods		
Know	215	**82,7**
Do not know	45	**17,3**
Total	260	**100**
Knowledge about the usefulness of using ARVs during pregnancy and during childbirth		
Know	200	**76,9**
Do not know	60	**23,1**
Total	**260**	**100**

III.2.4.3 Factors that influence HIV-positive women's knowledge of the importance of using contraceptive methods to reduce the risk of mother-to-child transmission

Age:

Among HIV-positive women who know the importance of using contraceptive methods to reduce the risk of mother-to-child transmission, 89.2% are 35 years of age or older and 75% are younger than 35.

Woman's education level:

For HIV-positive women who have completed elementary school and > 85.3% know the benefits of using contraceptive methods and for women who have attended primary school but did not finish and did not go to school, 77.7% know the benefits of using contraceptive methods.

There was a statistical association between the woman's knowledge of the importance of using contraceptive methods to reduce the risk of mother-to-child transmission of HIV and the woman's level of education (p=0.018).

Husband's education level:

For women whose husbands have attended primary school or less, 84.4% know the importance of using contraceptive methods and 71.4% of women who know this importance, their husbands have attended secondary school or more.

There was a statistical association between the wife's knowledge of the importance of using contraceptive methods to reduce the risk of mother-to-child transmission and the husband's education level (p=0.053).

Woman's profession:

For women engaged in other activities, 100% know the importance of using contraceptive methods, and for women engaged in household and agricultural work, 79.5% know it.

There was a statistical association between the woman's knowledge of the importance of using contraceptive methods to reduce mother-to-child transmission and the woman's occupation (p=0.012).

Marital status:

For women with a marital status other than married, 82.7% know the importance of using contraceptives and 82.6% of married women know the benefits of using contraceptive methods.

There was no statistical association between the woman's knowledge of the importance of using contraceptive methods to reduce the risk of mother-to-child transmission and marital status (p=0.637).

Parity:

Among women who know the importance of using contraceptive methods to reduce the risk of mother-to-child transmission, 85.7% have at least one child and 70% have no children.

There was a statistical association between the woman's knowledge of the importance of using contraceptive methods to reduce the risk of mother-to-child transmission and the woman's parity (p=0.000).

The elements described above are represented in Table 8.

Table 8: Factors that influence HIV-positive women's knowledge of the importance of using contraceptive methods to reduce the risk of mother-to-child transmission.

Variable	Workforce	of women who know the benefits of using contraceptives	Those who do not know any advantage	X^2	P	Decision
Age of the woman (in years)						
< 35	120	75(90)				
> 35	140	89,2(125)				
Total	260	82,6(215)		28,127	0,255	NS
Woman's level of education						
Primary attended but not completed + no school Primary	90	77,7(70)	22(20)	3,714	0,018	**
completed and beyond	170	85.3(145)	14,7(25)			
Total	260	82,6 (215)	17,3(45)			
Husband's level of education						
Primary education and less	225	84,4(190)	15,5(35)	3,704	0,053	*
Secondary education and above	35	71,4(25)	28,5(10)			
Total	260	82,6 (215)	17,3(45)			
Woman's occupation	220					
Household and agricultural work	40	79,5(175) 100(40)	20,4(45) 0(0)	5,165	0,012	**
Other **Total**	260	82,6(215)	17,3(45)			
Marital status						
Brides	115	82,6(95)	17,320)	2,544	0,637	NS
Other	145	82,7(120)	17,2(25)			
Total	260	82,6(215)	17,3(45)			
Parity						***
No children	50	70 (35)	30(15)	9,379	0,000	
At least one child	210	85,7 (180)	14,2(30)			
Total	260	82,6(215)	17,3(45)			

III.2.4.4 Messages received by HIV-positive women to avoid new pregnancies

215 women, i.e. 82.7%, received the messages during counseling to avoid new pregnancies being HIV positive, against 17.3% who did not retain any message. Thus, 40% received the message about the risk of contamination of the child during pregnancy/delivery and through breast milk, all three at the same time; 22.7% during delivery only, 20% on other themes, 11.2% on the risk of abortion and

6% were informed about the probability of maternal death.

Table 9 shows this.

Table 9: Messages received by HIV-positive women to avoid new pregnancies

Messages received	Workforce	Percentage
Remembered at least one message	215	82,7
Did not receive any messages	45	17,3
Total	**260**	**100**
Types of messages received :		
Contamination of the child during pregnancy/delivery and through breast milk	86	40
Contamination during delivery only	49	22,7
	24	112
Abortion		
Maternal death	13	6
Socio-economic problems	43	20
Total	**215**	**100**

111.2.5. Attitude of health care workers to key messages given to HIV-infected women on antiretroviral therapy during counseling to prevent further pregnancies.

Of the personnel interviewed, 40% were nurses, 31.4% were social workers, 20% were laboratory assistants and 8.5% were doctors.

All have a positive attitude about the messages to be given to HIV-infected women during counseling.

Table 10: Distribution of staff surveyed by their attitudes about regular messages given to HIV-infected women

Staff qualification	Workforce	Favorable attitude in percentage	Percentage of unfavorable attitude
Physician	3	100(3)	0(0)
Nurse	14	100(14)	0(0)
Laboratory assistant	7	100(7)	0(0)
Social	11	100(11)	0(0)
Total	35	100(35)	0(0)

111.2.6. Multivariate analysis for selected variables that showed a relationship

with the variable desire for motherhood after being on antiretroviral therapy

Calculation of the OR for the variables that showed a relationship with the dependent variable

We calculated 0R for the variables that showed a positive relationship with the "desire for pregnancy" variable, and these data are presented in Table 11.

Table 11: Data after OR calculation

Desire for motherhood after being on antiretroviral therapy according to	95% OR(CI)	P	Decision
Age of the woman (in years) <35 > 35	 1,011[0,637-1,092]	 0,017	 **
Parity At least one child No children	 [2,13[1,236-3,558]	 0,000	 ***
Contraceptive use Yes No	 0,870[0,279-2,746] 	 0,050 	 *

We then considered all independent variables that maintained a relationship with the dependent variable.

These are the age of the woman, parity and regular use of contraceptive methods.

All of these variables were then entered into a single equation, i.e., logistic regression, and the final model retained only two variables: parity and regular use of contraceptive methods.

Women who have not had a child have twice the desire for motherhood than women who have had at least one child.

In addition, women who regularly use contraceptive methods have a desire to have children that is almost 1 times higher than women who do not use contraceptive methods.

The elements described above are shown in Table 13.

Table 12: Data after logistic regression calculation

Variable: Desire for motherhood after being subjected to antiretroviral therapy as a function of:	OR(CI)	P	Decision

Parity		0.000	***
At least one child	2,15 [1,238-3,560]		
No children			
Use of contraceptive methods	0,877 [0,280-2,749]	0,051	*
Yes			
No			

CHAPTER 4: DISCUSSION

4.1. Frequency of pregnancy after knowledge of HIV status

4.1.1. Proportion of women who became pregnant after being informed of their HIV-positive status.

26.9% of the subjects in our study became pregnant after being informed of their HIV-positive status compared to 73.1% who did not become pregnant.

The results of our study are similar to those of a study conducted in the Caribbean where 182 HIV-positive women of childbearing age; 21.4% became pregnant after being informed of their positive HIV status(**25**).

In another study conducted in Zimbabwe among HIV-positive women of childbearing age, 31% of 52 women in the study became pregnant after knowing their HIV-positive status(**27**).

Thus, numerous studies in Europe, North America, Australia, the Caribbean and Africa have shown that HIV-positive women continue to conceive. Some do so voluntarily to satisfy their desire for motherhood and others for socio-cultural reasons (**27**).

4.1.2. Influential relationship between selected study variables and becoming pregnant after being informed of their HIV-positive status.

The educational level of the woman and her husband, the profession and the marital status of the woman do not influence the fact of becoming pregnant after knowing her HIV status. This could be explained by the fact that the desire for pregnancy among HIV-positive women is largely related to socio-cultural attitudes.

A similar situation was found in a study conducted in North America where the marital status of the woman and occupation did not influence HIV-positive women to continue to conceive, but rather, CD4 count and good health were the factors that influenced women to become pregnant (**28**).

Parity has an influence on becoming pregnant after knowing one's HIV-positive status (40% versus 23.8%).

A similar study in Rwanda on contraceptive use among HIV-infected women attending prevention of mother-to-child transmission (PMTCT) services found that women who had no children were likely to become pregnant after testing positive for HIV(**3**). These data suggest that young women with fewer children should be given special attention in reproductive health counseling.

A similar study of HIV-positive women of childbearing age in the United States showed that 12% of women who became pregnant after learning their HIV-positive status, 55% did not have children**(25).**

4.2. Proportion of HIV-positive women on antiretroviral treatment who want to have children in the future.

4.2.1. Proportion of women who want to have children in the future.

The proportion of women who want to have children in the future is 38.5% while 61.5% do not.

Work in other countries has also found lower proportions than in our study of HIV-positive women who intended to have new births after their HIV-positive diagnosis.

For example, studies in Uganda**(30)**, Zambia**(31)** and the United States of America**(32)** reported that 7%, 22% and 24% of HIV+ women on ARVs respectively wanted new births.

HIV-positive women who want more children need services that can educate and assist them in their choice.

The decision to consider a new pregnancy should be based on clear and adequate information.

4.2.2. Factors determining the desire for motherhood among HIV-positive women on ARVs according to reasons.

The first reason why women become pregnant despite their HIV status is the confidence that women attribute to ARVs (38%), followed by the HIV-negative status of the previous child (17.6%), then the refusal of the groom to use a condom and the desire of the husband to have a child (14.7%), the need for a replacement (8%), while the simple pleasure of having a child and the fear of the in-laws for each one of them (2.9%) come in last place.

In Zimbabwe, as in most other countries, the desire to have children is explained by both a need for affection and a need for financial security, especially if the woman is economically vulnerable.

Marriage is based on the hope of having children, especially if the husband's family has paid a dowry to the wife's family (**28**).

In a survey of 52 women in South Africa who wanted to become pregnant and were aware of their HIV status, the researchers also found 16 subsequent pregnancies, 9 of which were wanted**(29).**

Among the seven women who wanted their pregnancies, the medical history showed that they were sometimes willing to risk their own health to deliver a viable baby(**29**) .

4.2.3. Other factors that influence the desire for motherhood in HIV-positive women on ARVs

The age of the woman has a great influence on the desire of pregnancy in our study subjects. The subjects whose age is higher or equal to 35 years desire to have children than those whose age is lower than 35 years (39,2% against 37,5%)(p< 0,001).

Similar results were found by Lisann et al. in 2005 that women over 35 years of age had a greater desire for children than women under 35 years of age(**30**).

The level of education of the wife and husband, the profession, and the marital status do not influence the desire for motherhood in the subjects of our study.

On the other hand, parity (60% vs. 33% with p-value<0.05) and regular use (p<0.001) had a significant influence on the desire for pregnancy (39% vs. 37.9%) (p<0.001).

Women who do not have children want to have children much more than those who have at least one child.

These results are similar to those of a study done in Zimbabwe, where most of the women who wanted to have children were nulliparous (**29**).

Contrary results to ours were observed in a study done in the USA, among women who wanted to have children, 79% had at least one child(**17**). In fact, Thackway et al. in Australia in 1997, found that women who regularly use contraceptive methods have a greater desire to become pregnant than those who do not use contraceptive methods(**31**).

The wife's knowledge of the husband's HIV status did not influence the desire for pregnancy in the subjects of our study.

4.2.4. HIV-positive women's knowledge of the importance of using contraceptive methods and ARVs during pregnancy and childbirth to reduce the risk of mother-to-child transmission

4.2.4.1. HIV-positive women's knowledge of the usefulness of contraceptive methods to reduce the risk of mother-to-child transmission

The majority (83%) of the women in our study knew the importance of using contraceptives to reduce mother-to-child transmission.

4.2.4.2. HIV-positive women's knowledge of the usefulness of contraceptive methods to reduce the risk of mother-to-child transmission

The situation is almost identical for the knowledge of HIV-positive women about the usefulness of using ARVs during pregnancy and delivery, where 80% know this importance.

4.2.4.3. Factors that influence HIV-positive women's knowledge of the importance of using contraceptive methods to reduce the risk of mother-to-child transmission.

Age does not influence the knowledge of HIV-positive women on ARVs about the importance of using contraceptive methods to reduce the risk of mother-to-child transmission.

The level of education of the woman has an influence on the knowledge of HIV-positive women on the importance of using contraceptive methods to reduce the risk of transmission from mother to child. Women who had completed elementary school and above were slightly more aware of these benefits than those who had attended primary school but did not complete it and had no schooling (85.3% vs. 77.7%)(p <0.05).

The level of education of the husband has a small influence on the knowledge of HIV-positive women undergoing antiretroviral treatment about the importance of using contraceptive methods to reduce the risk of transmission from mother to child. Husbands who had attended primary school and less were more aware of these benefits than those who had attended secondary school and more (84.4% vs. 71.45)(p = 0.05).

This may be due to the simple lack of knowledge of some partners with any level of education about their wives' ability to control their contraceptive options or to discuss their use and access family planning services as a couple.

The woman's occupation influences HIV-positive women's knowledge of the importance of using contraceptive methods to reduce the risk of mother-to-child transmission.

Women engaged in other activities were more aware of these benefits than those engaged in household and agricultural work (100% vs. 79.5%) (p < 0.05).

The marital status of the woman does not influence the knowledge of HIV-positive women on ARVs about the importance of using contraceptive methods to reduce the risk of transmission from mother to child.

However, parity has an influence on the knowledge of HIV-positive women on ARVs about the importance of using contraceptives to reduce the risk of transmission from mother to child. Women who had at least one child were much more aware of these benefits than nulliparous women (85.7% versus 70%) (p <0.001).

This may be because HIV-positive women who have at least one child have already attended VCT/PMTCT and ARVS services and thus have been informed about contraception and its potential benefits.

The results of our study are similar to those of a study done by Birungi on the determinants of pregnancy desire among HIV positive women in Byumba District (2007) where the knowledge of HIV positive women on the benefits of using contraceptives was 62%(**2**) .

4.2.4.4. Messages received by HIV-positive women to avoid new pregnancies.

The results of our study show that 82.7% received at least one message during counseling to avoid new pregnancies compared to 17.3% who received no message.

In fact, HIV positive women received the message of the risk of contamination of the child during pregnancy/delivery and through breast milk (40%), followed by delivery only (22.7%), (20%) were advised on other topics, the risk of abortion (11.2%) and (6%) were informed about the probability of maternal death.

We found that a large number of women (17.3) did not receive any messages during VCT/PMTCT services and ARVs.

Even if these services are accessible, they are not always fully capable of meeting the needs of HIV-positive women, especially since nowhere was the use of contraceptive methods by the women in our study received as a message to avoid further pregnancies.

Similar results were found in a study of 69 HIV-infected women in the United States. It found that most participants acknowledged having access to methods of protection against pregnancy and sexually transmitted infections (STIs), but only half reported having received adequate family planning counseling (**33**).

In addition, a survey of 150 HIV-positive women

from an HIV/AIDS Center in Sao Paulo, Brazil, found that while clients were very satisfied with the services they received, they lacked information about reproduction and antiretroviral treatment to reduce the risk of mother-to-child transmission(**12**).

4.2.5. Attitude of health care workers toward key messages given to HIV-infected women on antiretroviral therapy during counseling to prevent further pregnancies.

All of the staff interviewed (100%) had a positive attitude toward giving messages to HIV-infected women during counseling.

In fact, 40% of the nurses are social workers, 31.4% are laboratory assistants and 8.5% are doctors.

37

CHAPTER 5: CONCLUSION AND RECOMMENDATIONS

CONCLUSIONS:

The results of our study on the determinants of desire for pregnancy among HIV-positive women on antiretroviral treatment in Rwamagana District show that our hypothesis is partially confirmed.

In fact, the proportion of repeat pregnancies as well as motherhood and desire for children among HIV-positive women undergoing antiretroviral treatment is high, as shown by the following:

1. The proportion of HIV-positive women who became pregnant after being informed of their HIV status was 26.9%.

2. The proportion of HIV-positive women undergoing antiretroviral treatment who wish to have children in the future is high, i.e. 38.5%. This desire is influenced by

- **Factors related to sociodemographic characteristics:**

S Age: Women aged 35 and over want to have children in the future more than women under 35 (39% versus 37.5%).

S Parity: nulliparous women are much more likely to want to have children in the future than those who have at least one child (60% vs. 34%), OR=2.13

S Regular contraceptive use: Women who regularly use contraceptives want to have children more than others who do not regularly use contraceptives (39% vs. 37.9%),0R=0.870

- **Other factors determining the desire for motherhood in HIV-positive women** on **ARVs**

A significant proportion of women, 65.3%, gave reasons for wanting to have children.

Indeed, the first reason is the confidence attributed to ARVs at 38%, followed by the HIV-negative status of the previous child at 17.6%, the husband's refusal to use condoms and the husband's desire to have a child at 14.7%.

However, HIV-positive women's knowledge of the importance of using contraceptive methods during pregnancy and childbirth to reduce the risk of mother-to-child transmission is satisfactory.

In fact, a significant proportion of the HIV positive women in our study (82.7%) know the importance of using contraceptives, while 76.9% know the importance of using ARVs during pregnancy and childbirth to reduce the risk of transmission from mother to child, which indicates a good level of knowledge about the usefulness of using contraceptives and ARVs during pregnancy and childbirth.

In addition, the attitude of health personnel towards the key messages given to women infected with HIV and on antiretroviral treatment during counseling to avoid new pregnancies is also satisfactory.

Indeed, the attitude of the health personnel is totally favorable or 100%, in the sense that they give messages that allow HIV positive women on ARVs not to become pregnant again.

Thus, these two elements (satisfactory level of knowledge on the part of mothers and satisfactory attitude on the part of providers), invalidate our hypothesis.

The results of this study allow us to identify the following weaknesses:

• The proportion of HIV-positive women on antiretroviral therapy who became pregnant after being informed of their HIV status is high

• The proportion of women who want to have children in the future is high, despite their HIV status.

• The majority of pregnancies among HIV-positive women after diagnosis of HIV infection were unplanned and these pregnancies are in part a direct consequence of unmet need for FP, highlighting the significant gap in family planning service provision for HIV-infected women/couples.

RECOMMENDATIONS :

The results of this study call for multiple actions to be taken, which is why we mainly recommend the following:

• Strengthen the integration of reproductive health and FP activities into HIV/AIDS services (PMTCT, HIV counseling and testing, and care of HIV-positive patients)

• Set up a follow-up program for HIV-positive couples who wish to have children to enable them to have pregnancies in the best conditions in order to reduce vertical transmission

• To awaken health personnel to be able to provide quality services to women and men who attend VCT, PMTCT&ARV services in order to allow them to have all the necessary information on the reduction of vertical transmission and the prevention of unwanted pregnancies.

•   To explore the influence of ARV treatment on the contraceptive practice and reproductive life of PLHIV.

•   Provide HIV-positive couples with all the necessary information on PMTCT, on the relationship between ARVs and pregnancy in order to significantly reduce transverse and vertical contamination.

•   Involve men more in FP programs, VCT/PTCT services, to help couples make joint reproductive health decisions.

BIBLIOGRAPHIC REFERENCE

1.Atangana MJ.Sexual 43pidemic of People living with HIV/AIDS in Younde,Cameroon.The XIII international AIDS conference,Durban,South Africa,July 9-14,2000

Birungi Francine: Determinants of the desire for pregnancy among HIV-positive women in Gicumbi, 2007

3.Birgit H.B van Bentema,Reproducyve choices among hiy-positive women soc.sci.Med.vol.46.No.2,pp171-179 Isabelle de Vincenzib,et al and the European Study on the natural History oh HIV infection in Women pregnancies before and after HIV diagnosis in European cohort of HIV-infected women.Aids 2000,p106

4.Bunnel RE,Yanpasarn S,and Kimarx PH,and HIV-1 seroprevalence among childbearing women in northern 43pidemic:monitoring a rapidly evolving epidepic.Aids 1999:13(4):509-515

5 .Chen JL, Phillips KA,Kanousse De, et al.Fertility desires and intentions of HIVPositive men and women.Family planning persepectives.2001;33(4):144- 152&165

6 .CDC,HIV testing among pregnant women, united states and Canada ,1998-2001,mortality weekly report,2002,51(45):1013-1016

7 Delvaux T,Elul B, et al.Evaluation of access to and utilization of prevention of mother to-child transmission(PMTCT) services in Rwanda,Ministry of Health.2007 Jan

9 .http ://www.actions-traitement.org/spip.article 634.juillet aout 2002

10 .James L.Chen,Kathryn A.Phillips, et al.Fertility desires and intentions of HIVpositive Men and Women.Family planning persepective 2001,32 July/August.

11 .Jones DL,Wess, wess SM,bhat GJ.,Bwaya V.influencing sexual practices among HIV-Positive Zambian women.AIDS care .2006 Aug;18(6):629-634

12 . Geneva: Joint United Nations Programme on HIV/AIDS, 2000.)

13 Nakayiwa S,Abang B.Packel P et al.Desire for Children and pregnancy risk behavior among HIV-infected men and women in Uganda.Aids behave 2006;10(suppl):S95-S104 Livinus 34

14 UNAIDS .Prevention of HIV transmission from mother to child: planning for programme implementation. Report from a meeting, Geneva, 23-24 March 1998 15. UNAIDS, WHO, Antiretroviral drugs and vertical transmission of HIV, Geneva 16.

15 Health Canada, HIV and AIDS in Canada: Surveillance Report to December 31, 2002.

16 .Stephanson JM et al;The study group for the medical reseach council collaborative study of women with HIV.The effect of HIV diagnosis on reproductive experience

19 .UNAIDS,WHO.AIDS 44pidemic update :December 2007(1Livinus)

20 Pregnancy and HIV/AIDS. volume 4. online. Available at: http://www.aidslaw.ca/francais/contenu/bulletinscanadien/ete99/f- pregnancy.htmailconsult on 12/1/2008

21 . WHO.UNFPA. Sexual and reproductive health of Women living with HIV/AIDS. Guidelines on care, treatment and support for women living with HIV/AIDS and their children in resource-constrained settings,Wold Health organization.2006 22.Winkison D,Abdool Karim SS,Williams B,Gouws E.High HIV incidence and prevalence among young women in rural south Africa: developing a cohort for intervention trials.J Aquir Immune Defic syndr 2000:23(5):405-409

23 Livinus Bangendanye: Use of contraception, desire for new pregnancies in HIV-infected women followed in the prevention of mother-to-child transmission of HIV (PMTCT) in Rwanda, January 2008 report.

24 Pregnancy and HIV: Monitoring the mother and child, available online at www.unimedia.fr

Joint United Nations programmes:AIDSepidemiupdate,Geneva: UNSAIDS/WHO,2007

25 Ariane Lisann bedimo.Ruth Bessinger, et al(1998).Reproductive choice among HIV-Positive Women.Autpatient program, department of medicine,Lousiana state university medical center, page 171-179

26 Green,G(1998): The reproductive careers of a cohort of men and women following an HIV-POSITIVE diagnosis. Journal of Biosocial Science,26,409-415 27.Feldiman R,Maposhere C.Voices and choices: a participatory reseach and advocacy study of reproductive health and rights of HIV positive women in Zimbabwe.The XIII international AIDS Confrence,Durban,South Africa,July 914,2000

28 Morrison C, Sekadde Kigondu C,Sinel S, et al.Is the IUD appropriate contraception for HIV infected women?presentation of thirteen th meeting of the international society for Sexualy transmitted Diseases Research,2005,July 11-14 2005

29 .

30 Galavotti C et al:(2000):Relationship between contraceptive method choice and

reproductive method, choice and beliefs about HIV and pregnancy prevention sex transmitted diseases, page 7-10

31 .Thackay et al.Fertility and reproductive choice in Women with with HIV-1 infection in Austraria.AIDS 1997,11:663-667

32 .Willson TE,Koening LJ,Walter E,et al.Dual contraceptive method use for pregnancy and desease prevention among HIV-infected and HV-uninfected women:The importance of an event-level focus for promoting safer sexual behaviors.Sex transim Deseases,2003

33 .Massad LS,Springera G,Jacobsona L, et al.Pregnancy rates and predictors of contraception of miscarriage and abortion in US women with HIV.AIDS.2004;18:28-286

APPENDICES

APPENDIX 1: QUESTIONNAIRE

Questionnaire number:/ /

Date of the survey:/   ///

Survey site: ....

A. Identification questions

NO	Questions and references	Coded answers	Jump
Q1.1	Age		
Q1.2	Level of education	1. No study done 2. Primary education attended and not completed 3. Primary education completed 4. Secondary education attended/completed 5. Higher education	
Q1.3	Your husband's level of education	1. No study done 2. Primary education attended and not completed 3. Primary education ends 4. Secondary education attended/completed 5. Higher education	
Q1.4	What is your profession	1. Household and agricultural work 2. Housework only 3. Paid work	
Q1.5	What is your husband's profession	1. Household and agricultural work 2. Housework only	

		3. Paid work	
Q1.6	What is your marital status	1. Single mother 2. Married 3. Widow 4. Divorced 5. Separate	
Q.1.7	How many children do you have?	1.0 2.1 3.2 4.>3	

B. QUESTIONS RELATED TO THE DESIRE TO BECOME PREGNANT

Q2.1.	How long have you known about your HIV status	1.< to 6 months 2.7 to 11 months 3. 12 to 23 months 4. 2 years and more 5. I don't know	
Q2.2	When did you know you were infected?	1.PMTCT 2.VCT 3.during an illness that makes suspect AIDS 4During the child's illness with AIDS	
Q2.3	Have you disclosed your HIV status to your husband/partner	1. Yes▶ 2.no 3. no answer	Q2.5
Q2.4.	Can you tell me why you did not notify your partner of your result?	1. Fear of being accused of being a source of infection 2Fear of being repudiated	

		3 Fear of being abandoned 4 .was not necessary 5 Fear that he will disclose the result 6 Other (please specify)	
Q2.5	Do you know your husband's HIV status	1. Yes 2. No	
Q2.6	How many pregnancies have you had after knowing your serology	1. 03.2 2. 14. >3	
Q2.7	How many children have you had since you have known your serology	1. 03.2 2. 14. >3	
Q2.8	Do you want to have children in the future?	1. Yes 2. No	
Q2.9	Does your husband/partner want it too?	1. Yes 2. No 3. I do not know 4. No answer	
Q2.10	How many children would you like to have?	1. 03.2 2. 14. >3	
Q2.11	Now that you know your serology, why do you want to have children?	I. I trust ARVs 2. I'm afraid of the in-laws 3. The previous child is negative 4 For the simple pleasure of having a child 5 If I don't give birth, others will laugh at me 6. My husband wants it 7. I need a replacement	

		8. My husband refuses to use a condom 9. I wasn't told it was bad 10. We are a discordant couple 11. I'm afraid of the in-laws 12. Other reasons(To be specified)	
Q2.12	Are you using a contraceptive method?	1. Yes▶ 2.no	Q2.14
Q2.13	If you are not using a contraceptive method, why?	1 ...Desire of pregnancy 2 Probability of having a child without infection through PMTCT or ARV use 3. Religious beliefs 4. I thought I was menopausal 5. My spouse refuses FP 6. Other reasons(Please specify)	
Q2.14	Do you intend to use contraceptives in the future?	1. Yes 2. No	
Q2.15	What are the benefits of using contraception in an HIV-positive woman?	1. I do not know 2. Avoid giving birth to a child who may be ill 3. Reinfection protection 4. No answer 5. Spacing out births 6.2,3,5	

C. ISSUES RELATING TO THE TAKING OF ARVs

Q3.1	How long have you been on ARVs?	Number of months.......	
Q3.2	Is there a benefit to using ARVs during pregnancy and delivery in HIV-positive women?	1. yes 2.no	
Q3.3	Where did you learn these benefits?	1. PMTCT 2. ARVs 3. VCT 4. Other (please specify)	
Q3.4	What are the benefits of using ARVs during pregnancy and childbirth in HIV-positive women?	1. I do not know 2. Protects the child against HIV 3. Protects the health of the mother 4. No answer 5. Other (please specify)	
Q3.5	What can women infected with HIV do to avoid infecting their offspring?	1 .taking ARVs 2 Breastfeeding the child for a short period of time (not to exceed 6 months) 3 Avoiding pregnancy/use of contraceptive methods	

D. QUESTIONS RELATED TO THE EVALUATION OF MESSAGES GIVEN TO POSITIVE WOMEN DURING COUNSELING BY HEALTH CARE STAFF

Q4.1	What is your qualification?	1. A doctor 2. nurse 3. a laboratory technician 4.Social 5.other (please specify)	
Q4.2	Have you provided pre- and/or post-	1. Yes	

	test counseling to HIV-infected women on the risks of HIV/AIDS on pregnancy, the life of the child and the mother in order to avoid new pregnancies?	2. No	
Q4.3	What are these risks given as messages?	1. Risk of contamination during pregnancy 2. Risk of contamination during delivery 3. Abortion 4. Maternal death 5. Contamination through breast milk 6. Other	
Q4.4	Are you in favor of the messages that are given during this counseling?	1. Yes 2. No	

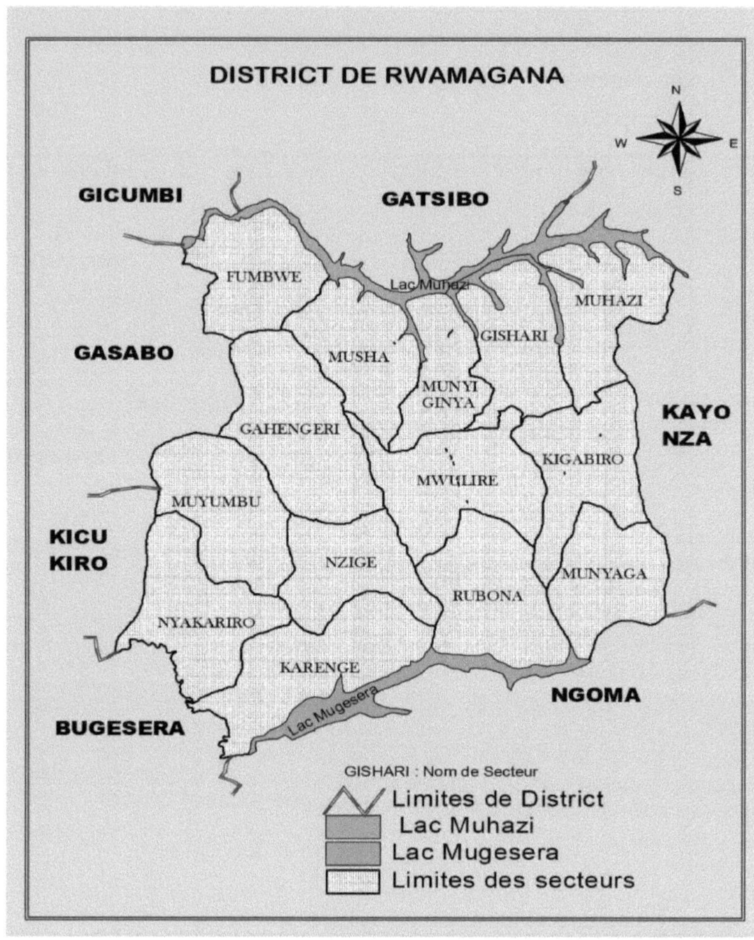

DISTRICT DE RWAMAGANA
N
W
E
S
GICUMBI
GATSIBO
FUMBWE
Lac Muhazi
MUHAZI
GASABO
MUSHA
GISHARI
MUNYI GINYA
GAHENGERI
KAYO NZA
KIGABIRO
MWULIRE
MUYUMBU
KICU KIRO
NZIGE
MUNYAGA
RUBONA
NYAKARIRO
KARENGE
NGOMA
Lac Mugesera
BUGESERA
GISHARI : Nom de Secteur
Limites de District
Lac Muhazi
Lac Mugesera
Limites des secteurs

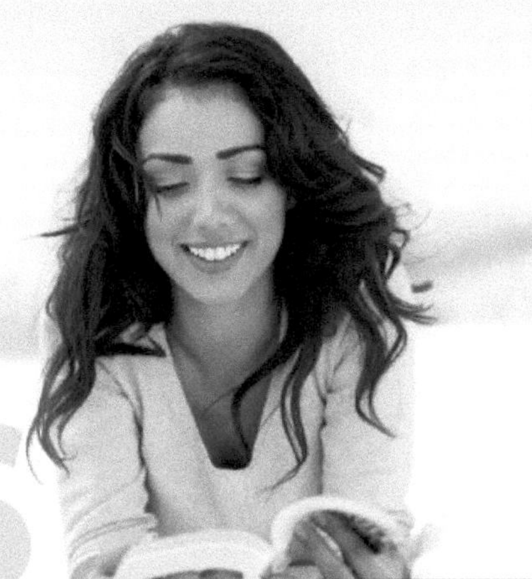

yes
I want morebooks!

Buy your books fast and straightforward online - at one of world's fastest growing online book stores! Environmentally sound due to Print-on-Demand technologies.

Buy your books online at
www.morebooks.shop

Kaufen Sie Ihre Bücher schnell und unkompliziert online – auf einer der am schnellsten wachsenden Buchhandelsplattformen weltweit! Dank Print-On-Demand umwelt- und ressourcenschonend produziert.

Bücher schneller online kaufen
www.morebooks.shop

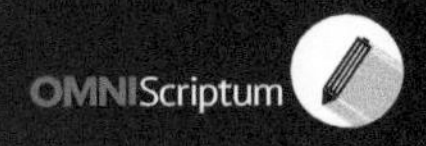

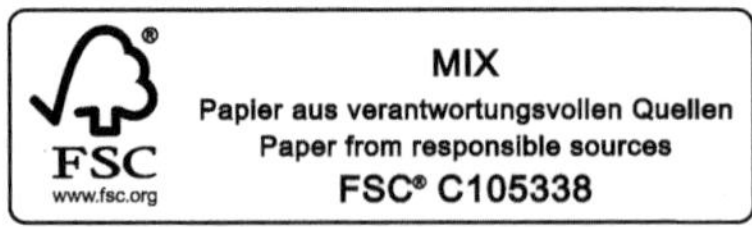

Printed by Books on Demand GmbH, Norderstedt / Germany